I0765995

RHINOPLASTY RECOVERY DIET

A Comprehensive Guide To Nutritional Support And Managing Discomfort And Nose Swelling For Vibrant Healing

DR LUCAS KAYCE

© [Dr Lucas Kayce] [2024]. All rights reserved.

Except for brief quotations included in critical reviews and certain other noncommercial uses allowed by copyright law, no part of this book may be reproduced, distributed, or transmitted in any form or by any means, including photocopying, recording, or other electronic or mechanical methods, without the publisher's prior written permission.

DISCLAIMER

This book about illness and nutrition is not meant to replace expert medical advice, diagnosis, or treatment; rather, it is meant purely for informational reasons. This book's content is founded on broad concepts and recommendations for managing diseases and nutrition.

Before adopting any major dietary or lifestyle changes, readers are recommended to speak with a qualified healthcare provider, such as a licensed physician or registered dietitian, especially if they have pre-existing medical concerns. Everybody has different health demands, so what works for one person might not work for another.

The use of the information provided in this book may have unfavorable repercussions or consequences, for which the author and publisher disclaim all liability. No disease is meant to be identified, treated, cured, or prevented by the information provided.

The book may include contain references to medical literature or research findings; however readers are urged to independently confirm this material and contact reliable sources.

It is important to remember that the fields of nutrition and medicine are always changing, and that new findings could have an impact on the advice offered in this book. As a result, readers are urged to keep up with the most recent advancements in healthcare and, when in doubt, seek professional counsel.

By reading this book, readers agree that they are in charge of their own health decisions and release the author and publisher from any liability arising from the use of the material in the book, whether direct or indirect.

TABLE OF CONTENTS

ABOUT THE BOOK

The "Rhinoplasty Recovery Diet" book provides a thorough overview of the postoperative treatment for rhinoplasty surgeries, which is frequently disregarded. This book explores the complex relationship between diet and the healing process, recognizing the importance of adequate nutrition during recovery and illuminating the critical role nutrition plays in ensuring the best possible outcomes following surgery.

The book gives a general summary of rhinoplasty in the introduction, highlighting both the procedure's transformative power and the special difficulties that come with recuperation. The principles of rhinoplasty are examined, along with the different surgeries and typical obstacles that people may face during their recovery.

The importance of nutrition in the healing process is the main topic. It clarifies the significance of eating a balanced diet and lists the particular nutrients—like protein, vitamins, minerals, and adequate hydration—that are essential for healing.

The book then walks readers through the preoperative period, providing dietary advice and useful stockpiling ideas for staple items.

Readers gain vital insights into managing the early postoperative period, switching to a soft diet, and introducing anti-inflammatory foods to minimize swelling as they work through. A road map for a gradual return to a regular diet, upholding a healthy lifestyle, and promoting scar healing through nutrition is provided by the long-term measures discussed.

While acknowledging that every person's path is unique, the book discusses typical obstacles that arise during the healing process and provides workable answers for changes in appetite, intestinal problems, and nutritional shortages. The book also includes a special chapter on consulting with a nutritionist, which highlights the value of getting professional advice.

"Rhinoplasty Recovery Diet" offers a planned and knowledgeable approach to postoperative nutrition, making it an essential tool for anyone having a rhinoplasty. This book gives readers the knowledge they need to maximize their recovery and get the most out of their rhinoplasty procedure by fusing medical insights with useful advice.

SYNOPSIS OF RHINOPLASTY

Rhinoplasty, also called a "nose job," is a surgical operation used to modify the nose's structure and form. This cosmetic procedure can fix breathing problems brought on by structural problems as well as address several concerns, such as nasal symmetry, size, and proportion.

Rhinoplasty has become increasingly popular due to its ability to improve both the functional and aesthetic aspects of the face. Reshaping the nasal bones, cartilage, and tissues requires precise surgical techniques, which frequently call for the assistance of a board-certified plastic surgeon.

There is historical proof that nasal reconstructive procedures were carried out in prehistoric societies, lending historical significance to the notion of rhinoplasty.

The process has been improved over time by developments in surgical methods and medical science, making it more accurate and safe. Nowadays, rhinoplasty serves as a way to improve the general well-being of people who may be facing functional difficulties as a result of their nasal structure, in addition to being a cosmetic procedure.

THE SIGNIFICANCE OF NUTRITION AFTER SURGERY

Now let's turn our attention to the postoperative phase. Nutrition plays a critical role in the healing process following surgical procedures like rhinoplasty. Postoperative care is equally important to promote good recovery and satisfactory results, even if the preoperative phase comprises extensive medical evaluations and conversations about the intended objectives. In this process, nutrition is essential since it helps the body heal damaged tissues, lower inflammation, and lessen the chance of problems.

Recognizing the body's heightened need for particular nutrients during the healing process is essential to comprehend the complexities of postoperative nutrition. For example, proteins are crucial for tissue regeneration and healing, which makes them the main component of a diet after a nose job. Furthermore essential for maintaining general health and facilitating the removal of postoperative toxins is enough water.

A diet high in nutrients and well-balanced is important for reasons beyond only physical recuperation. A sense of empowerment and control over one's recovery process can be fostered in patients having rhinoplasty through proper nutrition, which can have a good psychological influence. Patients are frequently advised to adhere to the dietary recommendations made by their medical providers, customizing their diet regimens to suit their particular postoperative requirements.

The complex procedure of rhinoplasty entails transforming the lives of people seeking both practical and esthetic advantages in addition to the physical aspects of the nose. Understanding the comprehensive nature of the process, postoperative care—especially about nutrition—becomes apparent as a critical factor in achieving favorable results. The best outcomes for individuals having rhinoplasty can only be achieved by integrating complete care—which includes both careful nutritional support and surgical expertise—as the field of plastic surgery continues to advance.

CHAPTER ONE

RECOGNIZING RHINOPLASTY

RHINOPLASTY: WHAT IS IT?

Rhinoplasty, sometimes referred to as a "nose job," is a surgical operation used to reconstruct or reshape the nose for either functional or cosmetic reasons. The Greek words "rhinos," which means nose, and "plastic," which means to shape, are the origin of the phrase "rhinoplasty". This cosmetic procedure can address several issues, such as modifying the nose's size, shape, and proportions, resolving breathing issues, or treating deformities brought on by trauma. A highly customized treatment, rhinoplasty involves the surgeon working closely with the patient to obtain the desired result while preserving the natural harmony of the facial features.

TYPES OF PROCEDURES FOR RHINOPLASTY

Rhinoplasty operations come in a variety of forms, each customized to meet the unique requirements and objectives of the patient:

• Cosmetic Rhinoplasty: This is the most popular kind, with an emphasis on improving the nose's aesthetic appeal. Cosmetic rhinoplasty can be used to change the nose's size, shape, or proportions in order to create a more harmonious and balanced facial profile. Surgeons employ a variety of methods, including tissue augmentation or removal, cartilage contouring, and nasal bone adjustments.

• Functional Rhinoplasty: Although aesthetic concerns are important, some people have rhinoplasty to address functional problems with the nose, like breathing problems brought on by structural abnormalities or a deviated septum. Functional rhinoplasty, which frequently entails modifications to the internal components of the nose, attempts to enhance airflow and relieve breathing issues.

• Revision Rhinoplasty: People may occasionally have a secondary rhinoplasty, also referred to as revision rhinoplasty, to rectify subpar outcomes from an earlier procedure or to address potential complications.

Because of scar tissue and changes to the nasal structure from the original treatment, revision rhinoplasty may provide greater challenges.

• Ethnic Rhinoplasty: This kind of rhinoplasty takes into accounts the distinctive facial traits and cultural preferences of patients from particular ethnic origins. The aim is to create a result that looks natural and harmonious in the context of the person's overall appearance, enhancing the nose while maintaining ethnic identity.

TYPICAL REHAB OBSTACLES

While everyone's recovery after rhinoplasty is different, the following typical issues are sometimes encountered throughout the healing phase:

• Swelling and Bruising: Following a rhinoplasty, swelling and bruising commonly occur around the eyes and nose. This normally goes away in the first week or two and is a normal reaction to surgical stress. These symptoms can be controlled with cold compresses, head elevation, and prescription medicine.

• Nasal Congestion: Swelling and transient changes to the nasal passageways may cause patients to have nasal congestion after rhinoplasty. At first, breathing via the mouth could be required. Saline sprays or nasal decongestants might be advised to relieve congestion.

• Pain and Discomfort: In the early days following a rhinoplasty, mild to moderate pain and discomfort are typical. The surgeon's suggested painkillers may help control this discomfort. Patients must adhere to postoperative recommendations, which include avoiding activities that may put undue strain on the healing nose.

• Removal of Splint and Dressing: Following surgery, patients may have a splint or dressing on their noses to support and safeguard the newly formed structures. Within the first week, these materials are usually removed, and patients may feel relieved as their nose starts to take on its new shape.

CHAPTER TWO

THE FUNCTION OF DIET IN HEALING

THE VALUE OF A BALANCED DIET

It is impossible to exaggerate the significance of a healthy diet in the healing process. A diet that is high in nutrients and well-balanced is essential for promoting the body's natural healing processes and facilitating faster recovery from disease, surgery, or accident. The vital components and energy needed for cellular repair, tissue regeneration, and general health restoration are provided by a balanced diet.

VITAMINS FOR REMEDY

Consuming enough high-quality protein is one of the mainstays of a diet aimed at healing. One essential food that helps with the production and repair of muscles, tissues, and organs is protein. People frequently have higher protein requirements during the recovery stage to aid in the healing process. Lean protein sources, such as chicken, fish, beans, and dairy products, can greatly aid in the healing process by enhancing overall strength and muscle integrity.

MINERALS AND VITAMINS

Apart from protein, vitamins and minerals are essential for promoting healing. These micronutrients participate in several metabolic reactions that are necessary for healing as cofactors. Vitamins like D, which is essential for healthy bones, and C, which is well-known for its function in the production of collagen, aid in the healing process as a whole. Similar to this, minerals like zinc and magnesium are essential parts of a diet focused on rehabilitation since they aid in immune system function, wound healing, and muscular contractions.

DRINKING WATER

Another essential component of diet during recovery is hydration. Water is a necessary nutrient that helps with digestion, nutrition transport, and temperature regulation, among other body processes. Maintaining optimal organ function and assisting the body in getting rid of waste materials is made possible by maintaining proper hydration. To promote healing, people in recovery should be mindful of how much fluid they consume and make sure they stay sufficiently hydrated.

A full recovery requires a well-balanced diet with a variety of nutrient-dense meals. Together, the vital vitamins, minerals, and antioxidants found in whole grains, fruits, veggies, and healthy fats help the body repair and rebuild itself. A balanced diet can also have a favorable impact on energy and mood, which helps support general well-being while in recovery.

Nutrition plays a complex role in healing, including the significance of a healthy diet, certain nutrients like protein, vitamins, and minerals, and keeping enough fluids in the body. The body's capacity to mend and recover can be greatly aided by a careful and balanced approach to diet, which will ultimately promote a quicker and more thorough restoration of health.

CHAPTER THREE

GETTING READY FOR RHINOPLASTY RECUPERATION

GUIDELINES FOR PREOPERATIVE NUTRITION

It's critical to concentrate on preoperative nutrition before rhinoplasty to make sure your body is ready for both surgery and recovery. Sufficient nutrition has the potential to facilitate the healing process, lower the likelihood of problems, and enhance the overall ease of recovery. It's crucial to eat a balanced diet full of vital nutrients like proteins, minerals, and vitamins. To customize your preoperative nutrition plan according to your unique health requirements, speak with your surgeon or a qualified dietitian.

Stressing the importance of eating a diet rich in fruits and vegetables can supply a variety of antioxidants that help strengthen the immune system. One important step in the healing process is reducing inflammation, which these antioxidants can aid with. Lean proteins found in fish, chicken, and lentils can also help with tissue healing and repair. Maintaining enough hydration is similarly vital; it can help remove toxins from the body and is necessary for optimal cellular function.

It is best to stay away from excessive alcohol and caffeine use as these substances might cause dehydration and disrupt blood coagulation. It's also critical to adhere to any special instructions your surgeon may have given you on fasting before surgery. By adhering to these preoperative dietary recommendations, you can help your body become stronger and healthier, which can facilitate a quicker recovery.

KEEPING UP WITH NECESSARY FOODS

Recovery from rhinoplasty takes more planning than just the day of the procedure, and having a kitchen well-supplied with necessary foods can make the recuperation process less stressful. Make nutrient-dense, easily digestible foods your priority to aid in your body's healing processes. Think about storing up foods like soups, broths, and soft fruits that don't require much chewing.

Foods high in protein, such as yogurt, eggs, and soft cheeses, can help rebuild tissue, and complex carbs and whole grains give you energy that lasts. When boiled or pureed into soups, fresh veggies provide essential vitamins and minerals. You may want to keep a variety of condiments and spices on hand to add appeal to your meals while you're recovering. That being said, you must speak with your surgeon regarding any dietary limitations or case-specific advice.

Think about keeping water alternatives handy in addition to solid foods. Plain water, electrolyte beverages, and herbal teas can all aid in preventing dehydration and enhancing general well-being.

To reduce anxiety and guarantee a smooth recovery following surgery, it is advisable to schedule and shop for these necessary foods well in advance of the procedure day.

TIPS FOR MEAL PLANNING

One of the most important aspects of getting ready for rhinoplasty rehabilitation is meal planning. During the first few days after surgery, meal preparation can be made easier and more manageable by keeping your diet simpler. To avoid spending a lot of time cooking while recovering, think about prepping and freezing meals. For a consistent supply of nutrients and to prevent overburdening your digestive system, choose smaller, more frequent meals.

To keep your guests interested and satisfied, incorporate a range of textures and flavors into your dishes. Foods can be blended or pureed; this is particularly helpful if chewing is painful during the early stages of recuperation. Ensure that your meals are well-balanced, with a combination of protein, carbohydrates, and healthy fats to support general health and healing.

It's vital to convey any dietary limitations or preferences to those aiding you during your recovery time, ensuring that your food plan fits with your individual needs.

CHAPTER FOUR

THE IMMEDIATE POSTOPERATIVE PERIOD

CLEAR LIQUID DIET

The immediate postoperative period is a vital time in the recovery process for persons who have undergone surgical procedures. During this time, patients are generally encouraged to follow a clear liquid diet as part of the gradual transition from fasting to regular eating. A clear liquid diet often contains fluids that are transparent and easily digestible, such as water, clear broths, fruit juices without pulp, and gelatin. This nutritional approach serves numerous functions, including limiting dehydration, delivering important nutrients, and allowing the digestive system to gradually restore its normal function.

Clear liquid diets, however limited in terms of variety, assist meet the patient's water demands while minimizing stress on the digestive system.

These easily digested fluids also aid in reducing problems such as nausea and vomiting, common postoperative concerns. The gradual reintroduction of solid foods often follows the clear liquid phase, allowing the gastrointestinal tract to adjust progressively to more complex dietary components.

MANAGING DISCOMFORT AND SWELLING

Managing discomfort and edema is a vital element of postoperative care. Surgical procedures can induce varied degrees of discomfort and swelling, which can influence the patient's general well-being.

Healthcare practitioners adopt a multimodal strategy to address these difficulties, sometimes combining drugs for pain management with efforts to minimize swelling. Non-opioid analgesics, such as acetaminophen or nonsteroidal anti-inflammatory medications (NSAIDs), are often used to ease pain, while localized treatments like ice packs and compression may be applied to minimize swelling in specific locations.

The efficient management of discomfort and swelling relies on a joint effort between healthcare practitioners and patients. Clear communication regarding pain levels and adherence to recommended drugs are critical for optimal pain relief. Additionally, patients are generally recommended to elevate the affected body regions and engage in moderate motions as tolerated to aid the reduction of edema. Physical therapy may also be prescribed to enhance mobility and encourage a faster recovery.

HYDRATION STRATEGIES

Hydration strategies play a vital role in the initial postoperative period, influencing the overall recovery process. Adequate hydration is required for several physiological activities, including circulation, organ function, and the elimination of waste materials from the body. Intravenous fluids may be delivered soon after surgery to ensure hydration and maintain electrolyte balance. As the patient transitions to oral intake, healthcare personnel often monitor fluid intake carefully, balancing the requirement for hydration with any restrictions imposed by the surgical procedure or the clear liquid diet.

Hydration measures extend beyond immediate postoperative care and are key components of the total recovery strategy. Patients are recommended to continue monitoring their fluid intake and balancing the consumption of clear beverages with water-rich foods to facilitate healing. Proper hydration not only benefits recovery but also helps prevent issues such as bladder retention and constipation, which can be prevalent following surgery.

The early postoperative period needs careful consideration of nutrition choices, pain management, and hydration measures to achieve a smooth healing process. The use of a clear liquid diet, appropriate treatment of discomfort and edema, and attentive hydration practices collectively contribute to maximizing the patient's recovery experience and enhancing overall well-being.

CHAPTER FIVE

TRANSITIONING TO A SOFT DIET

INTRODUCTION TO SOFT FOODS

Transitioning to a soft diet is a regular necessity for persons confronting various dental, gastric, or swallowing concerns. This dietary change entails picking foods that are simple to chew and swallow, relieving discomfort, and encouraging sufficient nutrition during recovery periods or continuing health issues. Soft diets can be various, allowing individuals to maintain a balanced and enjoyable eating experience while fitting their demands.

RECIPES AND MEAL IDEAS

Creating appealing meals on a soft diet demands a strategic approach to component selection and preparation methods. Soft meals don't have to be bland; instead, they can be tasty and nutritionally rich. Incorporating a diversity of textures and flavors is vital to keep meals interesting and delicious.

Examples of soft diet-friendly ingredients include cooked vegetables, tender meats, cereals, and well-cooked legumes. Experimenting with herbs, spices, and sauces can add richness to the whole dining experience.

SOUPS AND BROTHS

Soups and broths are basic components of a soft diet, offering both water and sustenance. Broths can be created from chicken, beef, or vegetables, and they serve as a base for numerous soups. Adding soft vegetables, such as carrots, potatoes, and squash, boosts the nutritional content while retaining a pleasing texture. Pureeing soups can further facilitate swallowing for persons with difficulties chewing. Cream-based soups, such as a smooth tomato bisque or a velvety broccoli cheddar soup, can also be excellent options for individuals on a soft diet.

PROTEIN-PACKED SMOOTHIES

Protein-packed smoothies are a wonderful way to ensure persons on a soft diet acquire essential nutrition.

Combining components like yogurt, milk, or plant-based alternatives with fruits, nut butter, and protein powders can produce delightful and gratifying beverages. Smoothies offer a simple approach to integrating critical vitamins and minerals while catering to the soft-texture requirement. Additionally, they may be adjusted based on particular taste preferences and nutritional demands, making them a versatile solution for any soft diet.

Shifting to a soft diet is a nutritional alteration that can enhance the quality of life for those experiencing specific health concerns. With ingenuity in the kitchen, one can produce a range of delicious and healthy dishes that fit the criteria of a soft diet. Whether through tasty soups and broths or protein-packed smoothies, soft meals may be both delightful and supportive of overall well-being.

CHAPTER SIX

INCLUDING ANTI-INFLAMMATORY FOODS

YOUR DIET TO LOWER SWELLING

Including items that reduce inflammation in the diet is a comprehensive way to support general health and control long-term inflammation in the body. Eating foods that are proven to minimize edema is an important part of this dietary regimen. These foods support the body's natural anti-inflammatory activities since they are frequently high in antioxidants, vitamins, and minerals.

Numerous fruits and vegetables are known to have anti-inflammatory qualities. Antioxidants called anthocyanins, which are abundant in berries like strawberries and blueberries, have been demonstrated to have anti-inflammatory properties. Rich in vitamins, minerals, and phytonutrients that boost the immune system and reduce inflammation are leafy greens, such as kale and spinach.

A diet rich in whole grains, including quinoa and brown rice, is also a great way to reduce inflammation. They include fiber, which helps lower inflammation in addition to facilitating digestion. Furthermore, fatty fish—such as mackerel and salmon—are great providers of omega-3 fatty acids, which have anti-inflammatory properties.

SUPPLEMENTS AND HERBAL TEAS

Another thing to consider for people who want to reduce inflammation is adding herbal teas and supplements. For example, curcumin, a substance with strong anti-inflammatory and antioxidant qualities, is found in turmeric. Incorporating turmeric into meals or drinking turmeric tea can be a tasty and nutritious method to reduce inflammation. Similar to this, ginger has anti-inflammatory properties and can be used in a variety of meals or drunk as a tea due to its unique flavor and possible health advantages.

Supplements such as fish oil-derived omega-3 fatty acids can strengthen an anti-inflammatory regimen even more. Before introducing supplements, it's important to speak with a healthcare provider to be sure they meet specific needs and don't conflict with prescription drugs already in use.

USING ANTI-INFLAMMATORY INGREDIENTS IN COOKING

Choosing carefully the culinary components to use when cooking with anti-inflammatory products promotes general wellness. For example, olive oil is widely used in Mediterranean cooking and is well known for having anti-inflammatory qualities. It has polyphenols and monounsaturated fats, both of which have been linked to decreased inflammation.

Commonly used aromatic components in many different types of cooking, garlic, and onions also have anti-inflammatory properties. They can be added to a wide variety of recipes to boost their nutritional content and flavor. Herbs such as oregano, thyme, and rosemary not only give food dimension but also have anti-inflammatory and antioxidant properties.

Adopting an anti-inflammatory diet entails choosing foods carefully that actively aid in lowering swelling and promoting general wellness. People can actively support a healthier and more balanced lifestyle by including a range of fruits, vegetables, whole grains, herbal teas, and supplements that reduce inflammation in their regular meals. Additionally, preparing food with anti-inflammatory substances can change the culinary experience, making it a nutritious activity for the body in addition to being delicious.

CHAPTER SEVEN

LONG-TERM DIETARY APPROACHES

RETURNING GRADUALLY TO A REGULAR DIET

A key component of long-term nutrition solutions is the gradual transition from any dietary restrictions or alterations back to a typical diet. This strategy is especially pertinent to people who have adhered to specific diets for weight control or medical purposes. Abrupt switches to a regular diet could be problematic for the metabolism and digestive system. Reintroducing different food groups gradually decreases the chance of nutritional imbalances and allows the body to acclimate. With the help of this methodical approach, people can better understand how their bodies react to various meals and adjust their diets for long-term health.

SUSTAINING AN INVIGORATING LIFESTYLE

A healthy lifestyle adoption and maintenance are closely related to sustainable long-term nutrition. A holistic approach goes beyond the restrictions of particular diets and includes regular physical activity, stress management, and sleep priority. Together with diet, these lifestyle choices promote general health. Frequent exercise improves muscular strength and cardiovascular health in addition to increasing metabolism. Stress-reduction strategies like mindfulness and getting enough sleep support hormonal balance and mental health. Together, these elements form a strong foundation for upholding a healthy lifestyle that accentuates and strengthens the advantages of a balanced diet.

NUTRITIONAL SUPPORT FOR SCAR HEALING

When it comes to scar healing in particular, nutrition is essential to the healing process. Giving the body the proper nutrients promotes tissue healing and reduces scarring. Collagen synthesis is a vital component of skin structure, and essential minerals like zinc, protein, and vitamins C and E are critical in encouraging its synthesis.

Fish and flaxseed, which are rich sources of omega-3 fatty acids, have anti-inflammatory properties that help reduce scar formation. Fruits and vegetables include antioxidants that help shield cells from oxidative stress and speed up the healing process. Another essential component for skin suppleness is adequate hydration. By including these nutrients in a long-term dietary plan, you can optimize scar healing and strengthen the body's innate healing abilities.

An all-encompassing long-term nutrition plan includes a gradual transition back to a regular diet, upholding a healthy lifestyle, and providing specialized nutritional assistance for particular health issues, such as scar healing. This strategy not only guarantees long-term well-being but also gives people the power to make educated decisions that suit their health objectives.

CHAPTER EIGHT

TYPICAL PROBLEMS AND THEIR FIXES

HANDLING SHIFTS IN APPETITE

Managing changes in appetite is a typical difficulty that people may face as a result of a variety of circumstances, including stress, hormonal changes, changing lifestyle choices, or medication.

It's critical to understand that changes in appetite are a normal aspect of life and may not always present an issue. But it's important to address these changes when they cause problems or lead to unhealthy eating habits.

Eating mindfully is one practical strategy. This entails being very aware of signals from the body regarding hunger and fullness, as well as responding to physical hunger rather than emotional ones when eating. Additionally, by balancing blood sugar levels and avoiding excessive hunger or overeating, sticking to a regular meal schedule might help regulate appetite.

Adopting a healthy, well-balanced diet is another important tactic. A healthy appetite can be maintained by consuming a range of nutrient-dense meals, such as fruits, vegetables, lean meats, and whole grains. Since dehydration can occasionally be confused with hunger, staying hydrated is also essential.

Seeking advice from a healthcare provider is essential when long-lasting changes in appetite are linked to underlying medical issues or pharmaceutical side effects. They can identify the underlying cause and suggest suitable interventions, such as individualized lifestyle modifications, hormone therapy, or prescription adjustments.

RESOLVING DIGESTIVE PROBLEMS

Many people worry about digestive problems because they can have a big influence on their quality of life. Bloating, gas, constipation, and diarrhea are common issues that are frequently caused by poor food choices, stress, or underlying gastrointestinal disorders.

One of the most important steps in treating digestive problems is making dietary improvements. Consuming a diet high in fruits, vegetables, and whole grains can help prevent constipation and encourage regular bowel movements. Probiotics support a healthy gut flora and may ease some stomach discomfort. They are present in meals like yogurt and fermented goods.

Staying hydrated is essential for preserving gut health. Maintaining a healthy digestive system, avoiding constipation, and ensuring optimal nutrient absorption are all facilitated by drinking enough water. However excessive intake of some irritants, such as alcohol and coffee, can worsen digestive issues, so moderation is advised.

It is essential to speak with a healthcare provider for a proper diagnosis and customized treatment options for ongoing digestive problems. Depending on a patient's needs, they could suggest testing to find underlying diseases, write prescriptions for drugs to treat symptoms or offer advice on particular dietary adjustments.

TAKING CARE OF NUTRITIONAL DEFICIENCIES

Deficits in nutrition can have a serious negative impact on general health and well-being. Fatigue, compromised immune system, and diminished cognitive function are just a few of the health problems that can result from consuming insufficient amounts of vital vitamins and minerals.

An important first step in addressing nutritional deficiencies is to diversify your diet by including a range of nutrient-rich foods. A wide range of vital nutrients can be included including fruits, vegetables, lean proteins, whole grains, dairy products, and dairy substitutes. Supplements may be considered for those with particular dietary needs or preferences, but to prevent overdosing, they should be used under a doctor's supervision.

Early detection of dietary deficits can be facilitated by routine blood testing to evaluate nutritional status.

CHAPTER NINE

HAVING A NUTRITIONIST CONSULTATION

WHEN TO LOOK FOR EXPERT ADVICE

Consulting a nutritionist becomes imperative when people have certain health issues or objectives that call for tailored dietary recommendations. Addressing pre-existing medical issues like diabetes, hypertension, or food allergies is one typical reason to see a nutritionist. These experts can create customized meal plans to successfully manage these diseases, guaranteeing that people get the right nutrition while meeting their medical requirements.

It can be beneficial for athletes and those aiming to achieve particular fitness objectives to speak with a nutritionist. These professionals may create individualized diet programs to stimulate muscle growth, improve general physical health, and maximize performance.

A professional's supervision is often necessary to achieve the ideal balance of macronutrients and micronutrients in sports nutrition due to its intricate nature.

Another important area where seeing a dietitian can be beneficial is weight management. A nutritionist may create long-lasting eating plans and offer evidence-based guidance to anyone trying to maintain healthy body composition, add muscle, or reduce weight. This entails learning about the person's metabolism, way of life, and preferences to design a strategy that will work over the long run while still being practical.

For those looking to adopt a better lifestyle, seeing a nutritionist can be helpful in addition to addressing specific health concerns or fitness goals. A nutritionist may provide insightful advice on portion management, balanced eating, and nutrient-dense food selections even in the absence of a specified health condition or fitness objective.

This preventive measure can lower the chance of developing health problems in the future and improve general well-being.

TAILORING A RECUPERATION DIET PLAN

Customization is essential when thinking about a recovery food plan to successfully handle individual demands and situations. A nutritionist designs a rehabilitation diet that fits each person's needs by taking into consideration variables including age, gender, activity level, and any pre-existing medical issues. A nutritionist may recommend nutrient-dense diets to a patient recuperating from surgery or illness to strengthen the immune system and promote healing.

Evaluating food preferences and lifestyle factors is another step in creating a personalized recovery diet plan. Together with the patient, a dietitian helps include foods that are sustainable, pleasurable, and helpful for healing. This guarantees that the patient is more likely to follow the food guidelines as directed, facilitating a quicker recovery.

Addressing any nutritional deficits that may have developed as a result of the disease or medical condition is an essential component of a personalized recovery diet plan. To close these nutritional deficits and advance general health, the nutritionist could suggest particular vitamins or dietary adjustments. Keeping an eye on things and adjusting as needed are essential components of the process because recuperation is frequently a dynamic process that calls for gradual diet plan revisions.

Seeing a nutritionist is appropriate for several circumstances, such as controlling medical conditions, reaching physical fitness objectives, or embracing a healthier way of life. Customization of recovery diet plans is necessary to meet specific needs and encourage the best possible recuperation.

www.ingramcontent.com/pod-product-compliance
Lightning Source LLC
Chambersburg PA
CBHW060813260726
48660CB00002B/927